The Sympathetic Nervous System and Hypertension

The Sympathetic Nervous System and Hypertension

Dr Michael Schachter
Senior Lecturer
Department of Clinical Pharmacology
Imperial College School of Medicine
St Mary's Hospital
London

MARTIN DUNITZ

The views expressed in this publication are
those of the authors and not necessarily those
of Martin Dunitz Ltd.

© Martin Dunitz Ltd 1997

First published in the United Kingdom
in 1997 by
Martin Dunitz Ltd
The Livery House
7– 9 Pratt Street
London NW1 0AE

Reprinted 1998, 1999

A CIP record for this book is available
from the British Library.

ISBN 1-85317-426-2

Printed and bound in Spain by Cayfosa

Contents

Preface

Hypertension is a very odd condition. It can hardly be called a disease, since it lacks not only a single recognized aetiology but even an unequivocal definition. It is a condition defined quantitatively, rather than qualitatively, leading to uncomfortable decisions for the clinician: is a systolic blood pressure of 161 mmHg 'abnormal', whereas 159 mmHg is 'normal'? Although the concept of total cardiovascular risk (with lipids, diabetes and smoking, among other factors, taken into account) makes this type of situation easier in one sense, it can also be regarded as a way of simply considering more parameters before making an arbitrary decision. A further peculiar feature of hypertension is the exceptionally large number of drugs used to treat it. All of these work in some patients and to some extent, but we know much less than we would like about the reasons when they do *not* . This has several practical consequences: many, probably most, hypertensive individuals take two or more drugs, and we are far from the situation where we can say that we have all the types of antihypertensive medication that we need to treat our patients. Finally, we have seen in the last couple of decades, as the number of effective agents has increased, that prescribing is distinctly susceptible to fashion and indeed to skilful marketing. At least in part this has been conditioned by shifting emphases on different theories of the aetiology of 'essential' hypertension. This has probably led to the neglect of some potentially useful therapeutic approaches. This short book focuses on one such area and tries to put it into the overall context of the management of this very common and very important condition.

A word, finally, about references. As in every other field of bio-medical activity the literature is enormous and growing rapidly. A huge reference list is very tedious for both author and reader, and probably of little real use to the latter. I have therefore cited a limited number of key primary sources but rather more secondary ones, which will give access to the literature for those interested in greater detail.

1. The Regulation of Blood Pressure — A Very Brief Overview

This chapter is a brief summary of our current under-standing of the mechanisms controlling blood pressure under physiological conditions. It emphasizes the predominant roles of the nervous system and the kidney. Nervous control has both short- and long-term components, whereas renal regulation is largely on a longer-term basis.

Given the crucial role of blood pressure in homeostasis it is hardly surprising that its regulation is a highly complex process, involving many mechanisms both for long-term control and for short-term responses to specific situations.

Central and peripheral nervous control

In the last 20 years we have acquired a reasonably coherent picture of the neural control of blood pressure, although much of the fine detail is still uncertain. A greatly simplified scheme is shown in Fig. 1. Some points need to be emphasized.

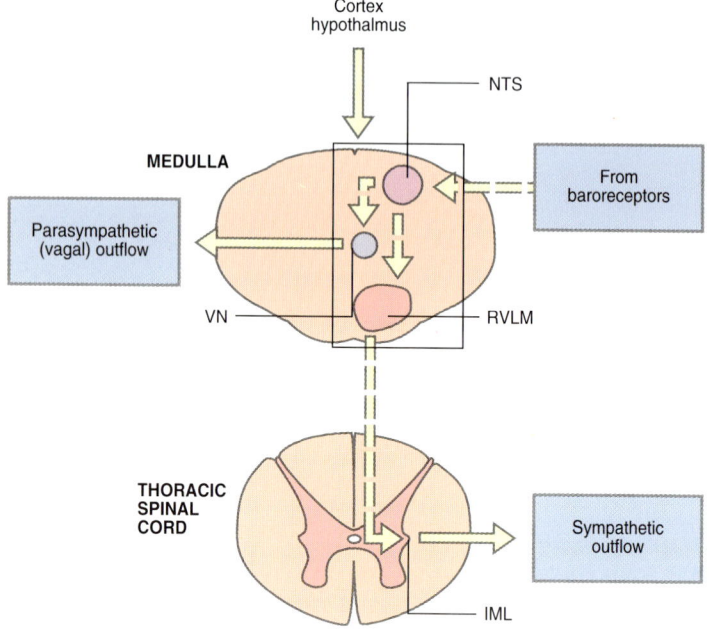

Figure 1
*Scheme of principal neural control mechanisms for the cardiovascular system.
NTS, nucleus of the tractus solitarius; VN, vagal nucleus; RVLM, rostral
ventrolateral medulla; IML, intermediolateral column.*

- The *sympathetic nervous system* is by far the most important effector
  pathway in blood pressure regulation. The vast majority of
  sympathetic fibres are vasoconstrictor, with noradrenaline
  (norepinephrine) as the principal peripheral neurotransmitter in the
  vascular wall; however, there are others, such as neuropeptide Y and
  adenosine triphosphate, but these have received little attention from
  a therapeutic standpoint

- The *ventrolateral medulla* (strictly the rostral ventrolateral medulla) is
  the principal pressor region in the brainstem, forming part of what is
  sometimes referred to as the vasomotor centre. It is a key component

in the baroreceptor reflex (see below) and its destruction causes the virtual abolition of sympathetic nerve discharge and a large fall in blood pressure. It is highly likely that this region contains neurones that are tonically (that is, constantly) active, and provide background stimulation for the preganglionic neurones of the spinal cord which connect to the ganglia in the sympathetic chain. The ventrolateral medulla therefore provides the central drive for vasoconstrictor tone

- The *dorsomedial medulla* (principally the *nucleus of the tractus solitarius*) is a depressor centre, inhibiting the output of the vasoconstrictor centre. Its destruction therefore leads to a sharp increase in blood pressure

- Many *higher centres* in the brain also have an input into blood pressure control. The most important are thought to be: the *hypothalamus*, where distinct areas have pressor or depressor effects; the *amygdala*, which is closely involved in emotional response, and where once again adjacent areas can have opposing effects on blood pressure; and several areas of the *cortex*

The central nervous system is particularly closely involved in the rapid alteration of blood pressure (almost always an increase) in response to various types of stress, of which one of the most fundamental and frequent is change of posture. This brings into play the best known cardiovascular homeostatic mechanism, the *baroreceptor reflex* (Fig. 2). Baroreceptors are nerve endings in arterial walls sensitive to stretch, and therefore to pressure. Although they are widely distributed, the most important are those in the aortic arch and near the carotid bifurcations. In principle these are simple feedback mechanisms (Fig. 3). The response of the system is very rapid, as is appropriate when posture is changed from a supine to a standing position; in this case the fall in blood pressure reduces discharge from the receptors, leading to *increased* sympathetic activation, increased blood pressure following widespread vasoconstriction and also increased heart rate. The baroreceptor reflex considerably dampens the short-term variability

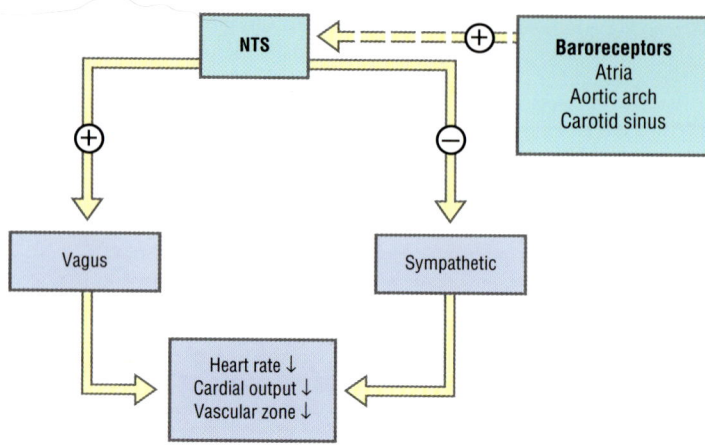

Figure 2
The baroreceptor reflex, illustrating the effect of increased activation of baroreceptors. NTS, nucleus of the tractus solitarius.

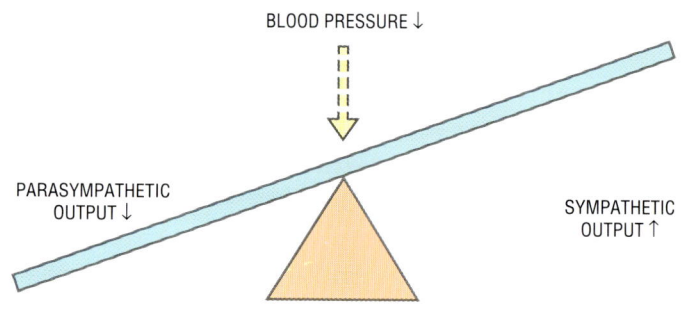

Figure 3
Simplified view of autonomic response to fall in blood pressure.

of arterial pressure and is therefore regarded as a pressure 'buffer' system. Other forms of stress, such as exercise, also usually lead to increased blood pressure subsequent to generalized vasoconstriction, while local factors (see page 7) can promote regional vasodilatation, for instance in active skeletal muscle.

Renal and hormonal factors

The nervous system plays a very prominent role in the long-term regulation of arterial pressure, largely by the modulation of sympathetic vasoconstrictor tone, and is of pre-eminent importance in short-term adaptation. By contrast, the kidney is very largely involved in longer-term regulation of blood pressure, especially in relation to body sodium and water homeostasis. This point is illustrated in a very simplified form in Fig. 4. The point of equilibrium may be 'reset' if renal function is impaired, thereby leading to increased blood pressure: the curve therefore shifts to the right. Similarly, expanded extracellular volume leads generally to increased blood pressure, but in this case the set-point moves *along* the curve. In most circumstances in humans salt intake is the principal determinant of extracellular volume and therefore a major factor in the modulation of blood pressure.

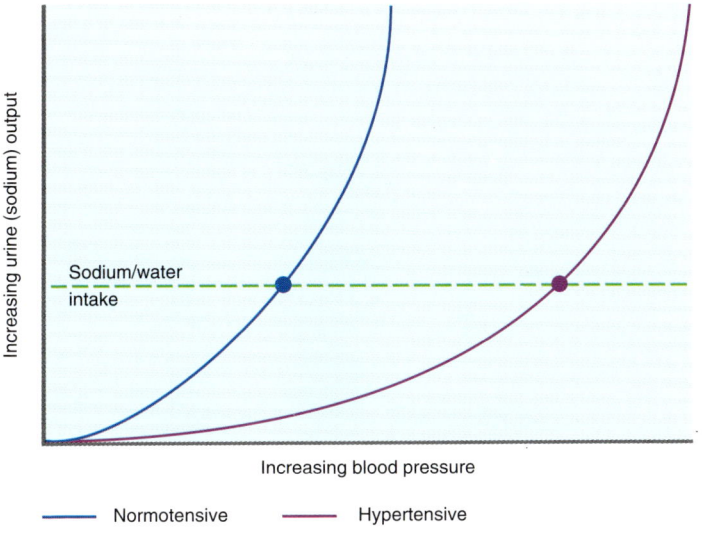

Figure 4
Scheme of blood pressure regulation by the kidney, illustrating the concept of the 'set point' and its resetting in hypertension.

The kidney is also the focus of one of the principal hormonal blood pressure regulators, the *renin–angiotensin–aldosterone (RAA) system*. This is summarized schematically in Fig. 5. The system responds to stress fairly rapidly, but not with the imme-

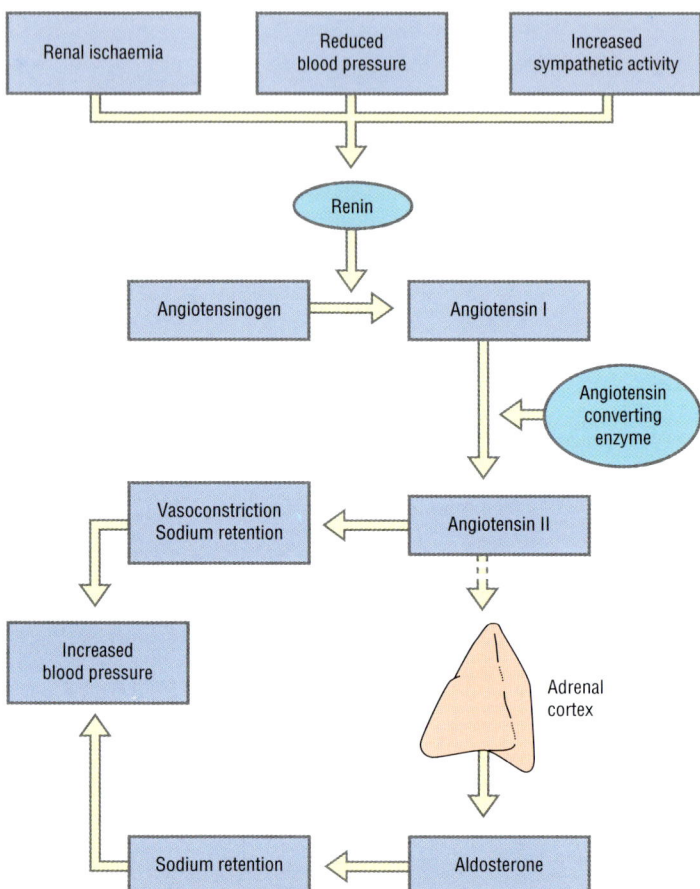

Figure 5
The renin–angiotensin–aldosterone system.

diacy of the sympathetic nervous system. Its ultimate purpose is the retention of sodium and water and therefore the maintenance of arterial pressure in the face of stresses such as haemorrhage. Angiotensin II has direct salt-retaining effects within the kidney but is also a very potent vasoconstrictor, so increasing blood pressure by at least two mechanisms. Further, it reinforces these effects by stimulating secretion of the sodium-retaining hormone aldosterone. It is not surprising that this system has become a paramount target for antihypertensive therapies in recent years.

Other *hormonal influences* will not not be discussed in any detail. Kinins, such as *bradykinin*, are powerful vasodilators which are thought to have a mainly local effect on blood flow. However, it is widely thought that increased levels of these peptides play a role in the antihypertensive action of the angiotensin-converting enzyme inhibitors, as well as in some of their unwanted effects (see page 39). *Corticosteroids* have a critical role in the maintenance of blood pressure, especially under conditions of stress: this is partly through an effect on sodium handling but this is not a complete explanation.

Local vascular factors

Kinins are not the only examples for which the distinction between local and systemic effects is less than clear-cut. This is particularly prominent for two endothelium-derived agents: *nitric oxide* (the formerly elusive endothelium-derived relaxant factor) and *endothelin*, a peptide which usually acts as an extremely potent vasoconstrictor. There is no doubt that both of these regulate blood flow and vascular resistance locally, but their systemic importance is more controversial. However, there is now evidence that systemic inhibition of nitric oxide synthesis does raise arterial pressure, and also some findings supporting a role for endothelin in maintaining elevated blood pressure. Whether deficient nitric oxide or excessive endothelin are actually significant aetiological factors in hypertension remains, nevertheless, highly questionable.

2. Mechanisms of Hypertension — A Jigsaw with Gaps

There is still no clear understanding of the cause of so-called 'essential' hypertension. Many theories have been proposed, involving the nervous system, the kidney, circulating factors and the interactions of these with each other and the environment. It is highly unlikely that a single gene abnormality will prove to be a major factor in the great majority of cases.

The underlying causes and mechanisms of essential hypertension — itself a name strongly suggestive of ignorance! — continue to arouse a remarkable degree of controversy. Much of the argument has indeed been less than dispassionate. There is, however, no dispute that the determinants of blood pressure are:

- cardiac output

- peripheral vascular resistance

This is usually expressed as:

> blood pressure = cardiac output x peripheral resistance

Hypertension is a reflection of *increased peripheral resistance* because of either an *absolute* increase in resistance or a *relative* increase with respect to cardiac output. The question, therefore, is: what is the underlying cause (or causes) of this alteration?

Only a small minority of cases of hypertension can currently be classified as secondary — between 5 and 15%, depending particularly on the age of the population concerned: the likelihood of an identifiable cause is greater in the young population, in which essential hypertension is uncommon. The principal causes of secondary hypertension are listed in Table 1. Even in these circumstances the precise mechanism by which blood pressure is raised is sometimes poorly understood.

Increased renin secretion	Renovascular disease Renin-secreting tumours
Increased adrenocortical hormones	Primary hyperaldosteronism (Conn's syndrome) Deoxycorticosterone excess (11β-hydroxylase deficiency) Corticosteroid excess (Cushing's syndrome, primary or secondary)
Increased catecholamines	Phaeochromocytoma
Drugs or other substances	Steroids Liquorice (in large quantities!), Carbenoxolone Sympathomimetics
Other causes	Pregnancy-related hypertension (including pre-eclampsia) Coarctation of the aorta

Table 1
Causes of secondary hypertension.

There is much greater difficulty in defining what happens in 'primary' hypertension. Few would doubt that this is a multifactorial condition, but there are widely different views on what constitutes the fundamental abnormality. The following are the principal *types* of hypothesis currently under discussion, but note that several are not mutually exclusive, and interactions are highly likely:

- Hypertension is primarily a disorder of the *central nervous system* and specifically of *sympathetic regulation*. This will be discussed in detail in the following section

- Hypertension is the result of an interaction between *environmental factors*, notably *high salt intake* and *psychosocial stress*, with each other and with the individual's genetic tendency to hypertension

- Hypertension is a *renal disorder*, specifically associated with *abnormal sodium handling*. This obviously may be related to the second hypothesis, above

- Underlying any or all of these hypotheses, as already indicated, is the question of *genetic predisposition*

- It is widely believed that, in a substantial minority of patients, hypertension forms part of a *metabolic syndrome arising from insulin resistance* (Fig. 6): that is to say, inadequate glucose uptake in response to insulin, particularly in skeletal muscle. Characteristically these patients are middle-aged males with, in addition to hypertension, upper body obesity, non-insulin-dependent diabetes and dyslipidaemia. This syndrome will be discussed further in Chapter 3

- Hypertension is characterized by changes in *vascular structure and function* throughout the circulation. There has been extensive discussion as to the importance of these changes — particularly in the microvasculature — in the pathogenesis of hypertension. Put simply, are they cause or consequence?

These concepts will be discussed below, but the list is very far from being exhaustive.

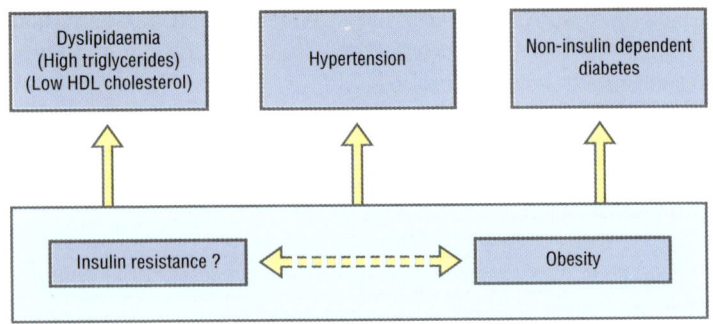

Figure 6
The concept of the insulin resistance syndrome (metabolic 'syndrome X').

Other theories have included: *abnormal handling of calcium ions; deficiency of adrenomedullin*, a circulating endogenous depressor compound; *excessive generation of vascular free radicals*, leading to degradation of nitric oxide and hence impaired vasodilatation; and *intrauterine growth retardation*, associated with abnormal development of the microvasculature. Detailed consideration of these is far beyond the scope of this book, but its lack does not imply any negative assessment.

Environmental factors (especially salt)

It is unlikely, although not inconceivable, that a single environmental factor might be enough to make someone hypertensive. More plausibly, several factors may interact with an underlying genetic tendency to produce hypertension. Much attention has focused on the role of dietary *salt* (in other words, *sodium*). Indeed, this topic has produced decades of controversy, some of it verging on the irrational. There is strong epidemiological evidence, notably from the INTERSALT study, that *population* blood pressure correlates positively with salt intake. These collective data are composed of the very varied response of individuals to increased salt intake — although even the definition of 'increased' is disputed. The methods used to define 'salt sensitivity' in individuals have varied greatly between researchers, and have often involved detecting reductions in blood pressure following salt restriction rather than increases produced by salt loading. Salt-sensitive patients, as well as normotensive controls, have shown a significant though usually modest fall in blood pressure on salt restriction.

Several factors appear to be associated with salt sensitivity:

- *race*: salt sensitivity is significantly increased in black hypertensive individuals (at least in the USA)

- *age*: there appears to be greater salt sensitivity with increased age

- *weight (?)*: although relationship between weight and salt sensitivity is inconsistent, weight loss in the obese seems to reduce salt sensitivity

- *family history*: most investigators have concluded that there is greater likelihood of salt sensitivity in the families of established hypertensive individuals

There has been an even greater variety in the mechanisms suggested to explain this phenomenon:

- *renal function*: reduced glomerular function is generally associated with increased salt sensitivity. Some evidence also suggests that salt-sensitive individuals may have an abnormal response in terms of altered renal blood flow. However, there has been much greater interest in a more active role for the kidney in mediating the effects of 'excess' salt. This has followed two main lines of enquiry, as discussed on page 14

- *insulin sensitivity*: as indicated previously, in certain populations of hypertensive individuals there is reduced responsiveness to some peripheral actions of insulin. However, not all studies have shown an association between salt and insulin sensitivity

Cont'd.

- *ion transport*: it has been suggested that abnormal salt sensitivity may form part of a generalized abnormality of transport reflected in all cells. It is not clear what the molecular basis of the underlying basis might be

- *endothelium-derived mediators*: recently it has been suggested that nitric oxide or endothelin may have a role in determining salt responsiveness

- *sympathetic nervous system*: many but not all groups have suggested a link between excessive sympathetic activity and enhanced salt sensitivity

The role of the kidney

From a historical perspective, the role of the kidney has attracted more attention than any other in hypertension research. Two main approaches require particular consideration: one of these is widely but not unanimously accepted. The importance of the second, the RAA system, is beyond doubt, at least in many instances of secondary hypertension.

The circulating sodium transport inhibitor (?)

The essential features of this theory, originating from the work of de Wardener, are summarized in Fig. 7. The vast literature on this subject includes many instances of apparent identification of the inhibitor. It has been suggested that it is of low molecular weight, and a cardiac glycoside-like agent similar to ouabain, or even ouabain itself. As the figure indicates, an incidental effect of such a compound — or compounds — would be an increase in vascular tone as an indirect result of increased intracellular sodium leading to raised levels of intracellular calcium. The relationship of this factor (if it actually exists) to the kidney is, as one might anticipate, also controversial:

- Is there a primary defect in the kidney, with reduced ability to excrete a sodium load ? It has already been noted that impaired sodium excretion is believed to be associated with an exaggerated pressor response to salt

- Does the increased concentration of the circulating pump inhibitor itself constitute the primary abnormality?

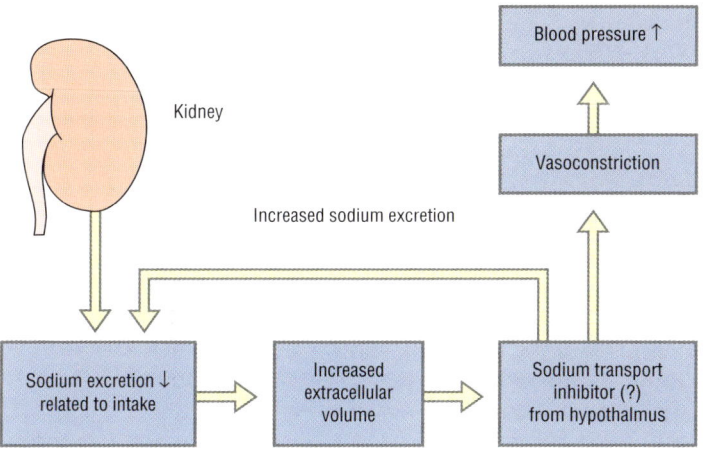

Figure 7
The role of the hypothetical sodium transport inhibitor in the pathogenesis of hypertension.

The relevance of these mechanisms in the overwhelming majority of hypertensive individuals remains very much open to question.

The renin—angiotensin—aldosterone system

In the context of secondary hypertension the most prominent role of the RAA system is in renovascular disease. Reduced perfusion of one or both kidneys is the trigger for the activation of the system. In most cases the diminished perfusion is due to narrowing of renal arteries on one or both sides. This is due in most instances to atherosclerosis or, in younger patients, to fibromuscular dysplasia. Although in many instances improved perfusion (by surgery or angioplasty) will normalize the bio-chemical abnormalities and the blood pressure, this does not necessarily occur, especially in the context of atheromatous disease. It is presumed that this is because of poorly reversible changes in the peripheral vasculature (see below).

Genetic factors

It was recognized many years ago that essential hypertension was most unlikely to be due to a single-gene abnormality. Little progress was made until the development of the techniques of molecular genetics, and even now our understanding of the problem remains rudimentary. There is evidence that there may be some linkage between essential hypertension and variants of the angiotensinogen gene, but so far this explains only a small proportion of the variance of the blood pressure. The genes for several rare types of Mendelian forms of hypertension have, however, been identified (for instance, glucocorticoid-remediable hypertension, due to inappropriate secretion of aldosterone which can be suppressed by glucocorticoids). All the genes so far identified which have a specific blood-pressure raising or lowering effect act on the RAA system or on other aspects of renal salt and water handling. One possible, and not too surprising, outcome of current genetic research may be the finding that essential hypertension is not attributable to a single gene: it is highly probable that it is due to an interaction of genotype and environment.

Vascular changes — primary or secondary?

Structural changes in the heart and vasculature have been recognized as long as hypertension itself. The whole of the vascular tree is affected in some way, but the critical changes occur in the small arteries/large arterioles where the largest pressure drop occurs. In these vessels there is an increase in the media/lumen ratio, which can occur in one of three ways (Fig. 8):

- *hypertrophy*: increase in the size but not the number of vascular smooth muscle cells

- *hyperplasia*: increase in number but not size of the smooth muscle cells

- *remodelling*: increase in neither cell size nor cell number: rearrangement of cells around a smaller lumen (i.e. overlapping)

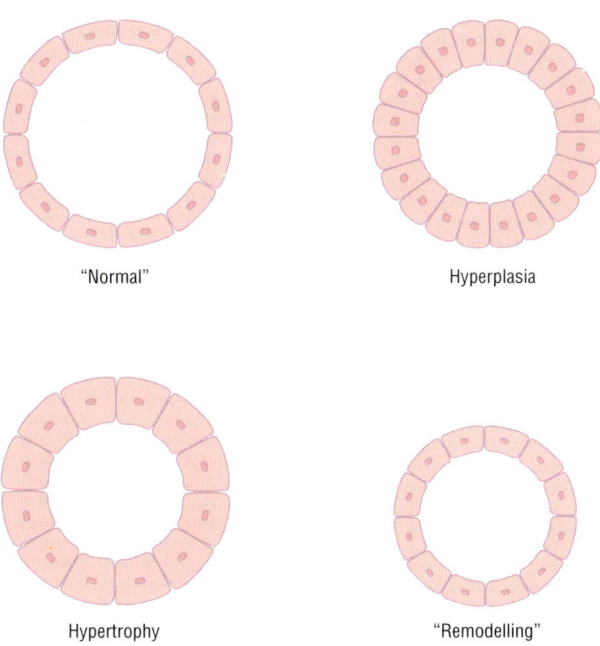

"Normal"

Hyperplasia

Hypertrophy

"Remodelling"

Figure 8
Alterations of the media/lumen ratio in blood vessels, particularly resistance arteries. Terms as defined in text.

The relative importance of these mechanisms is uncertain in animal models of hypertension and even more so in humans. Current concepts attribute a greater role to the third option, though in fact a mixture of all three may occur. In any case, there is *increased sensitivity to vasoconstrictors* and usually *reduced sensitivity to vasodilators*, specifically if these are endothelium-derived (although there are some divergent views on these points). Further downstream in the vascular tree there is *capillary rarefaction*.

The presence of the above features is almost universally accepted, but there is less agreement on their role in pathogenesis. Several possibilities exist:

- *primary changes in the resistance vasculature* (involving one or more of the above possibilities) producing increased peripheral resistance; such changes might relate to a generalized cellular abnormality, possibly involving membrane transport (see above)

- *secondary adaptive changes* due to pre-existing elevation of blood pressure

- a combination of these processes

A synthesis of these views has been proposed by Folkow in Sweden and Lever in Scotland. Their proposals are summarized in Fig. 9. The nature of the original vasoconstrictor stimulus is usually unknown, but sympathetic overactivity is one obvious candidate. Factors contributing to, or amplifying, structural change have not been definitely identified but there is no shortage of potential growth modulators (Table 2). The consequences of this are not merely academic, since it seems highly probable that long-term changes in vascular structure, however they may occur, are among the factors that can make drug withdrawal difficult or impossible in hypertensive patients.

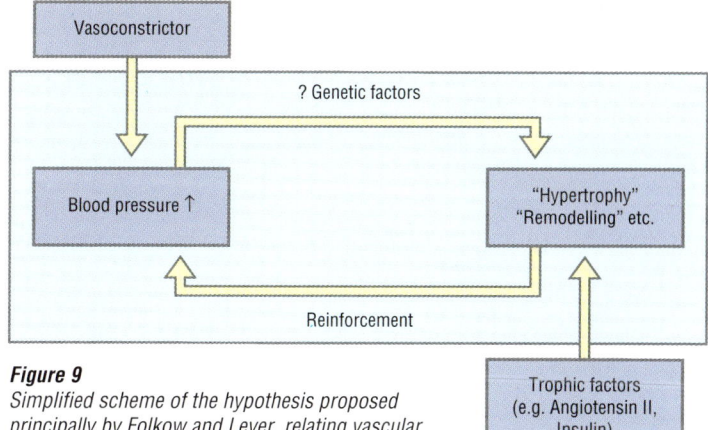

Figure 9
Simplified scheme of the hypothesis proposed principally by Folkow and Lever, relating vascular structure to the development of hypertension.

Growth promoters	Growth inhibitors
Platelet-derived GFs	Transforming GFs beta
Fibroblast GFs	Atrial natriuretic peptides
Epidermal GFs	Interferon gamma
Insulin-like GFs	Nitric oxide
Interleukins	Prostacyclin
Thrombin	Heparan/Heparin
Endothelin	
Angiotensin II	
Vasopressin	
Noradrenaline	
Serotonin	
Thromboxane	

GF, growth factor

Table 2
Potential growth modulators for vascular smooth muscle cells.

3. The Brain and the Sympathetic Nervous System

Overactivity of the sympathetic nervous system may play a significant contributory role in many patients with hypertension. This may be particularly so in young people with borderline hypertension, in patients with insulin resistance and in those with visceral obesity: there is very substantial overlap in the last two categories.

Essential hypertension

Most people would intuitively link 'stress' of a psychosocial nature with rises in blood pressure in the short term and, if biomedically trained, would attribute a major role to the sympathetic nervous system in bringing this about. However, to extend this line of thinking to *chronic* hypertension is not as simple as it might seem. There are two principal reasons for this: the complexities involved in assessing autonomic function in humans, or indeed in any intact animal; and the fact that autonomic activity is not constant during the evolution of hypertension. Although it will not be discussed in detail, it should be noted that there is a general reciprocal relationship between sympathetic and parasympathetic tone: some evidence suggests that the latter may predominate in determining heart rate, but not blood pressure. This section briefly considers the techniques available for the assessment of sympathetic tone and the evidence implicating this system in the pathophysiology of hypertension.

Assessing sympathetic function

It must of course be borne in mind that there is no single method for adequately quantifying a complex function such as this. However, the following complementary approaches all have a useful place, and are relevant to the subsequent discussion:

- *plasma catecholamine assay*: this obviously measures only the catecholamines cleared in the plasma rather than those metabolised in situ, and therefore only a small fraction of the total; these levels can reflect acute responses to stimuli, but for the same reason are highly variable

- *urinary catecholamine assay*: this is a more integrated measurement, usually covering a 24-hour period, but nonetheless suffers from the drawback that, again, only a very small percentage of released catecholamines is cleared by the kidneys

- *measurement of regional noradrenaline release*: this is an accurate estimate of catecholamine release from a region or organ, but often requires complex and invasive technology

- *measurement of noradrenaline turnover*: this may give an accurate picture of catecholamine release but may be invasive to some extent as well as needing complex calculations

- *direct sympathetic microneurography*: this is a direct estimate of sympathetic nerve activity, which may be representative of overall sympathetic tone. However, it is technically difficult to perform

- *spectral analysis of heart rate and blood pressure*: this can yield information about the relative activity of the sympathetic and parasympathetic systems, but is very significantly influenced by end-organ responsiveness

Borderline hypertension and sympathetic overactivity

From the use of these techniques and other approaches, it has been found that there are several types of evidence implicating the sympathetic nervous system and its regulation in the development of primary hypertension.

Several studies have noted that there is a distinct population of patients with borderline to mild hypertension (the *hyperkinetic state*, found in about 30–40% of the total) with the following characteristics:

- they are young (less than 40 years old)

- they are more often male

- they have high cardiac output

- their basal heart rate is also increased

Most of these individuals eventually develop established hypertension, presumably in the context of the adaptive vascular changes mentioned above. As this occurs, evidence of sympathetic overactivity becomes less marked, with normalization of both cardiac output and heart rate. Interestingly, in most instances when first characterized these individuals had higher blood pressures in the clinic than at home (the so-called 'white coat' effect. In these 'hyperkinetic' patients increased blood pressure and heart rate can be reduced by autonomic blockade, strongly suggesting a neurogenic cause for the abnormalities. This group of patients also had raised plasma noradrenaline levels. Regional studies indicate a selective activation of the sympathetic nervous system, involving the heart, kidneys, and skeletal muscle, but *not* the liver and mesenteric circulation. In keeping with this it has been reported that in these patients stress may induce greater kidney vasoconstriction than in normotensive subjects. Many but not all studies indicate that this group has exaggerated pressor responses to mental stress and some forms of exercise. It has been proposed that psychosocial stress, such as migration, may interact with increased salt intake to stimulate sympathetic activity and raise blood pressure. For instance, many villagers from rural Kenya became hypertensive within weeks of moving to Nairobi, with alteration in their diet and drastic changes in their lifestyle and environment.

The specifically renal consequences of sympathetic activation need to be emphasized:

> • vasoconstriction within the kidney increases sodium retention
>
> • the vascular effect, by reducing renal perfusion, promotes the release of renin and therefore activation of the RAA system
>
> • sympathetic nerve activation will *directly* stimulate renin release

It is also worth comment that this emphasizes how closely interrelated all these regulatory systems are in reality. It may often be convenient to speak of 'renal' and 'neurogenic' mechanisms but in practice it may be difficult or impossible to consider these in isolation.

If established hypertension does occur, the patient's haemodynamic state alters, as shown in Fig. 10. There is a transition from a high cardiac output state with apparently normal peripheral resistance to an apparently normal cardiac output state with high peripheral resistance. The *apparent* normality should be stressed: in the first instance the peripheral resistance is in fact *relatively* increased in the context of the increase in cardiac output; in the second the normal cardiac output may disguise a fall in stroke volume compensated for by increased heart rate.

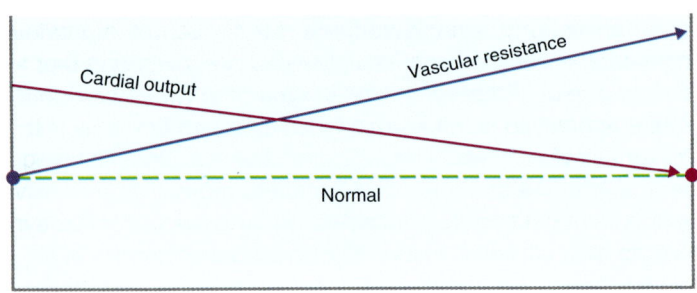

Figure 10
Changes in haemodynamics associated with transition from borderline to established hypertension.

Several questions arise from these concepts, particularly:

- how many patients diagnosed at the time when they already had *established* hypertension were previously borderline hyperkinetic hypertensives?

- is there one underlying cause for the sympathetic overactivity or are there multiple possibilities?

- are there any other types of patient in whom such overactivity may play a significant role?

There are at present no clear-cut answers to these questions, which in fact are closely interlinked, as the subsequent discussion will show.

Causes and consequences of increased sympathetic activity

The cause of the increased sympathetic drive in the hyperkinetic young hypertensive patient is not understood. However, there is another group of hypertensive patients in whom such a neurogenic abnormality probably plays a prominent role in pathophysiology. They have been mentioned in the previous section: the patients with *insulin resistance syndrome* (sometimes unhelpfully called metabolic syndrome X). The incidence of the syndrome is not known but it has been suggested that about half of all patients with hypertension fall into this category. It is also interesting to note that first-degree normotensive relatives of patients with hypertension and the metabolic syndrome are also likely to show insulin resistance.

Given that the syndrome is a valid entity, new questions arise:

- what are the mechanisms linking the components of the syndrome with insulin resistance?

- is the sympathetic nervous system likely to be involved?

At first sight the answer to the first question is not at all obvious. Insulin resistance is associated with hyperinsulinaemia, but giving normal individuals insulin infusions certainly does not raise blood pressure in the short term and may do the opposite. A plausible explanation is that the link is through activation of the sympathetic nervous system (Fig. 11). This in turn may be

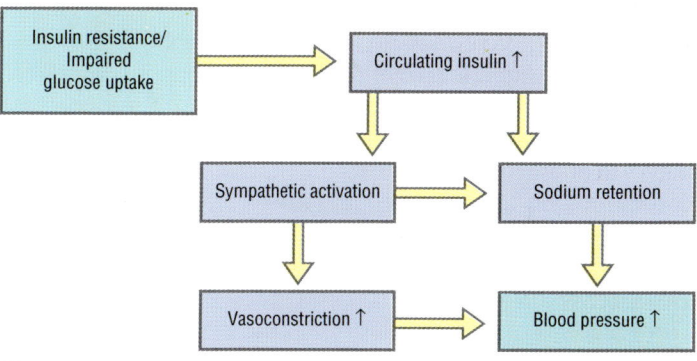

Figure 11
Potential mechanisms by which insulin resistance may be a causative factor in hypertension.

mediated through the action of insulin on a specific region (the ventromedial) of the hypothalamus, leading to disinhibition of sympathetic drive. There is certainly evidence that hyperinsulinaemia, with maintenance of normal blood glucose levels, does increase activity in sympathetic nerves, but the site of the interaction is unclear.

However, there is a contrary view, which is summarized in Fig. 12. It proposes that insulin resistance is *secondary* to hypertension, of whatever origin that may be. As always with chickens and eggs, it is not easy to resolve which of these comes first.

Obesity and the sympathetic nervous system

The link between hypertension and obesity is universally recognizd by clinicians. Upper body or 'central' obesity is of particular significance. Very frequently obese hypertensive patients can be included in the insulin-resistance metabolic syndrome but the question arises as to whether there is a specific link between obesity and raised blood pressure. Once again, the evidence is contradictory. Although some researchers have reported that insulin and body mass index are independent determinants of sympathetic activity, others have failed to find any connection. The balance of opinion does, however, favour some sort of close link between these variables and increased sympathetic activation in the obese. Figure 13 is based on one possible scheme. It may be that insulin is *not* an obligatory link between obesity and sympathetic overactivity and hypertension, but other alternatives shown (notably leptin) are equally speculative at present.

Secondary hypertension

Of the many possible causes of secondary hypertension listed in Table 1, only two will be considered here:

- phaeochromocytoma

- renovascular disease

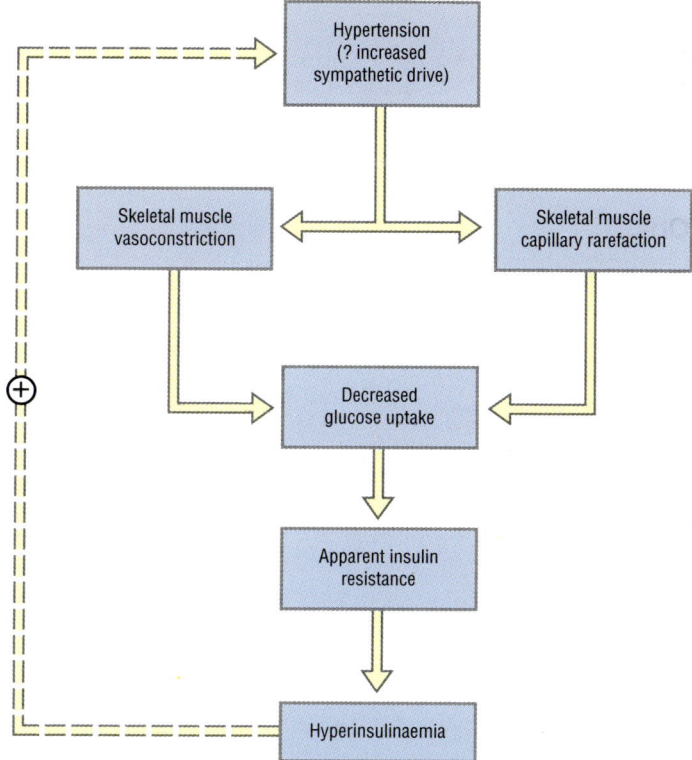

Figure 12
Alternative hypothesis, with insulin resistance as consequence rather than cause of hypertension.

Phaeochromocytomas are tumours of the so-called chromaffin cells found in the adrenal medulla and elsewhere in the sympathetic system. They secrete catecholamines, particularly

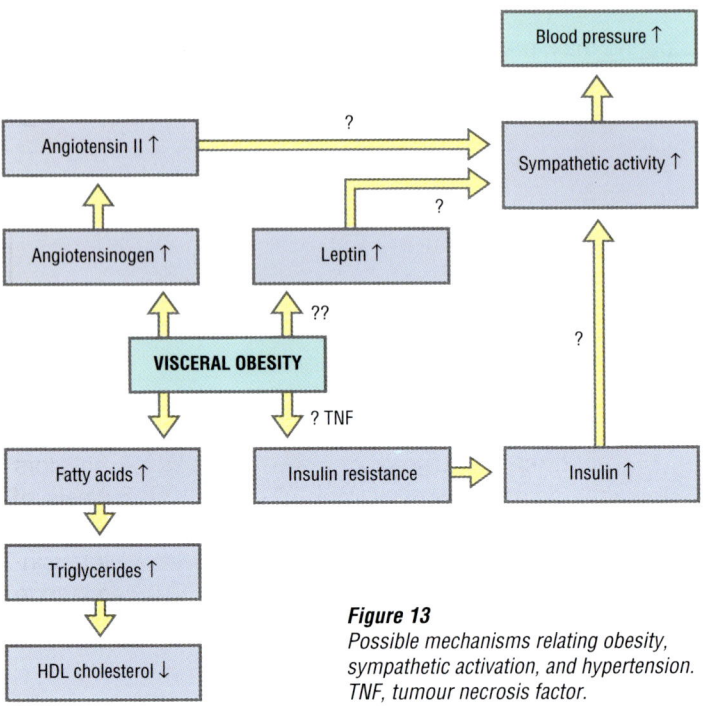

Figure 13
Possible mechanisms relating obesity, sympathetic activation, and hypertension. TNF, tumour necrosis factor.

noradrenaline, sometimes in very large quantities. They are characteristically associated with paroxysmal and often dangerously severe hypertension: however, sustained hypertension may also occur. Associated symptoms, such as palpitations, sweating, and anxiety, are those one would expect from sympathetic hyperactivity, in this case caused by circulating hormones rather than the sympathetic nervous system itself.

Renovascular disease usually includes stenosis of one or both of the renal arteries. In young people, particularly women, fibromuscular hyperplasia is the most common cause, whereas in older patients it is more commonly due to atheroma. The consequence of renal hypoperfusion is activation of the RAA system: local or systemic increases in plasma renin activity are a diagnostic feature of this condition. Angiotensin II is believed to be the main pressor component of the system, raising blood pressure by several mechanisms:

- direct vasoconstriction

- sodium retention by direct renal actions and by stimulating aldosterone secretion

- increasing sympathetic activation, by increasing noradrenaline release from nerve endings (and possibly by a central effect)

The sympathetic nervous system is therefore activated under these conditions, and angiotensin converting enzyme inhibitors can counteract this process by inhibiting the synthesis of angiotensin II. However, the overall effect may be harmful in these patients, since renal perfusion may be angiotensin-dependent, so that reduced levels of the peptide can lead to impaired renal function in the affected kidney(s) and even to renal failure.

4. Treatment of Hypertension — Central, Peripheral, or Both?

There are an extraordinary number of treatments available for lowering blood pressure, with many mechanisms of action. Most recent developments have focused on drugs acting on the peripheral vasculature but there is long experience with centrally acting agents. There are strong arguments for not neglecting these in considering the management of the hypertensive patient.

This section certainly is not a comprehensive overview of antihypertensive treatments. It is merely an attempt to put into context the means currently available, and a brief summary of their mechanisms (as far as they are understood) and their main advantages and drawbacks. The classes of antihypertensive drugs are listed in Table 3 and the main types of non-pharmacological interventions are listed in Table 4. As is shown, the majority of these drugs have a predominantly peripheral and vascular site of action.

'First-line' drugs

Diuretics	*Thiazides*
	Potassium-sparing
Beta-blockers	*Without vasodilator activity*
	With vasodilator activity
	with alpha$_1$-blocking properties
	with intrinsic agonist activity
	with other vasodilator activity
Calcium channel blockers	*Dihydropyridines*
	Others
	verapamil
	diltiazem
ACE inhibitors and receptor antagonists	angiotensin converting enzyme inhibitors
	angiotensin receptor (AT$_1$) antagonists
Alpha$_1$- blockers	

Other antihypertensive drugs

Centrally acting drugs	reserpine
	methyldopa
	clonidine
	moxonidine
Adrenergic neurone blockers	
Vasodilators with various mechanisms of action	diazoxide
	hydralazine
	minoxidil
	sodium nitroprusside (intravenous only)

Table 3
Antihypertensive drugs available in the UK (early 1997).

Weight loss	Magnesium supplementation*
Reduced salt intake*	Stress management
Reduced alcohol consumption**	– relaxation therapy
Exercise (aerobic)	– meditation
Potassium supplementation*	– yoga
Calcium supplementation*	

* several combinations reported
** in individuals with high initial intakes — may be closely related to weight

Table 4
Non-pharmacological treatments in hypertension.

Diuretics (especially thiazides)

Mechanism of action

It is ironic that, although thiazide diuretics are among the longest established and most extensively tested antihypertensive drugs, we still have a very poor understanding of their mechanism of action. As might be expected, they produce both volume depletion and sodium loss at first, accompanied by a fall in peripheral resistance (sometimes briefly preceded by an increase) and cardiac output. With chronic use (6–8 weeks or more) the reduction in peripheral resistance and increased sodium excretion persist, but cardiac output and blood volume gradually return to pretreatment levels. It is far from clear what is happening at this point but sodium depletion is probably crucial. A direct vasodilator effect is also possible but difficult to demonstrate.

Advantages

- very good evidence of efficacy and long-term reduction in stroke and cardiovascular events

- low cost

- convenient dosage regime

Disadvantages

- potential metabolic abnormalities: hypokalaemia and hyponatraemia, hyperuricaemia, impaired glucose tolerance, worsening lipid profile, hypomagnesaemia (these can be minimized by low doses and hypokalaemia specifically by concurrent potassium-sparing drugs such as amiloride)

- may cause postural hypotension

- may cause sexual dysfunction, especially in men

- rare liver, bone marrow, and skin toxicity

Beta-blockers

Mechanism of action

Once again, the exact mechanism of action of these drugs is uncertain, but the general view is that reduction in blood pressure is associated with diminished cardiac output in the presence of peripheral resistance which may actually increase in *absolute* terms. In drugs with partial agonist activity (so-called intrinsic sympathomimetic activity, or ISA), such as pindolol, there may be some fall in peripheral resistance and a less marked drop in cardiac output. Some other beta-blockers have more pronounced vasodilator activity from alpha-adrenergic blockade or direct action on smooth muscle (these include labetalol and celiprolol). The ultimate outcome in terms of blood pressure is much the same, resulting from a *relative* fall in peripheral resistance (Fig.14). Beta-blockers also cause a reduction in renin secretion, which can contribute significantly to blood pressure reduction in patients with high-renin hypertension. It is worth noting that in these patients, contrary to statements in most textbooks, the hypotension can be very abrupt.

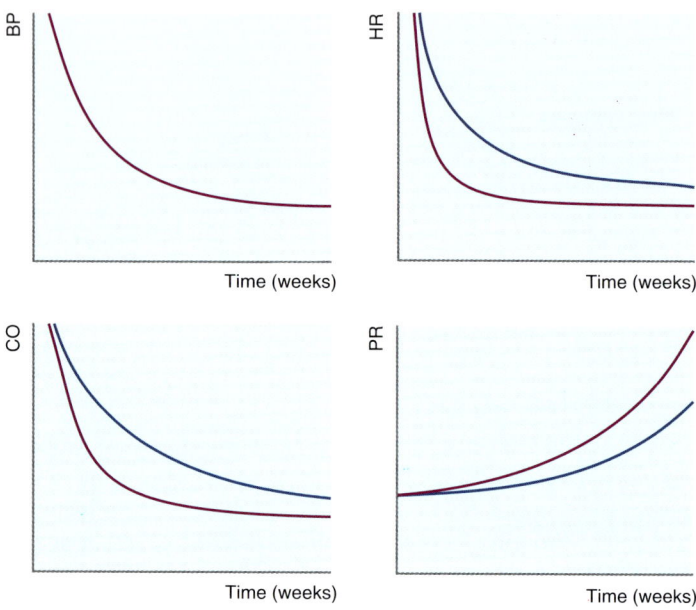

Figure 14
Chronic cardiovascular effects of beta-blockers, with (upper curve) and without (lower curve) sympathomimetic activity. BP, blood pressure; HR, heart rate; CO, cardiac output; PR, peripheral resistance.

Advantages

- long-term efficacy and clinical benefits well proven in trials

- useful in patients with co-existing angina

- usually simple once-daily dosing

Disadvantages

- can cause excessive slowing of heart rate, including heart block

- can precipitate heart failure because of inhibitory effect on cardiac contraction (negative inotropy)

- can cause dangerous bronchospasm in asthmatic patients

- may cause deterioration in peripheral vascular disease (probably only important for small vessel disease)

- can worsen lipid profile and insulin sensitivity (less marked in drugs with ISA or alpha-blocking properties)

- may decrease awareness of hypoglycaemia in diabetics

- can cause sleep disturbance, including nightmares

Calcium channel blockers

Mechanism of action

This is a heterogeneous group of drugs with differing properties, as shown in Table 5. Nonetheless, as far as their hypotensive effect is concerned it is likely to be the vascular effect that is crucial, with inhibition of calcium entry into blood vessels, reducing tone and hence peripheral resistance.

Advantages

- short-term efficacy good (note that there are *no long-term data on clinical outcome* for antihypertensive drugs apart from the older centrally acting drugs — reserpine and clondine —diuretics and beta-blockers)

- may be useful in angina (especially those that are not dihydropyridines)

- few absolute contraindications (e.g. safe in asthma)

- simple dosage regimes

Disadvantages

- may cause flushing, headache, ankle oedema (especially dihydropyridines)

- may cause reflex sympathetic activation secondary to vasodilatation (especially short-acting dihydropyridines), with increased heart rate — possible long-term adverse effects on cardiac events and mortality?

- may cause bradycardia, impaired left-ventricular function (especially those that are not dihydropyridines)

- rare gum hyperplasia (particularly dihydropyridines)

- possible increased risk of cancer (highly unlikely)

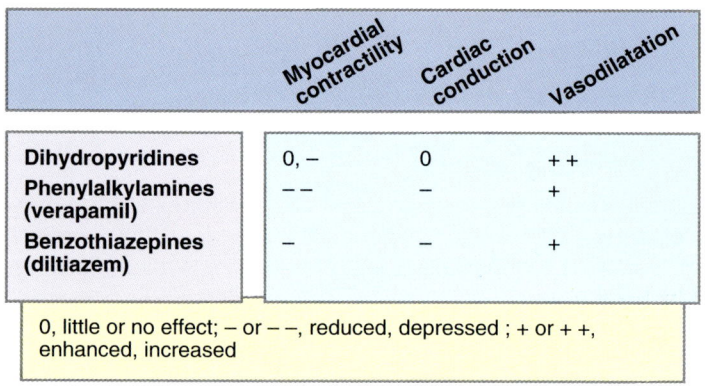

	Myocardial contractility	Cardiac conduction	Vasodilatation
Dihydropyridines	0, –	0	+ +
Phenylalkylamines (verapamil)	– –	–	+
Benzothiazepines (diltiazem)	–	–	+

0, little or no effect; – or – –, reduced, depressed ; + or + +, enhanced, increased

Table 5
Properties of different classes of calcium channel blockers.

Angiotensin converting enzyme (ACE) inhibitors and angiotensin receptor antagonists

It has already been noted that angiotensin II can raise blood pressure by several mechanisms, including the potentiation of sympathetic action. It is therefore not surprising that inhibition of angiotensin II formation, or antagonism of vascular angiotensin II receptors (the AT_1 subtype), will lower blood pressure in circumstances when there is high renin activity, even though total and uninterrupted blockade of angiotensin II synthesis may not be required. Interestingly, these drugs are also effective in some patients in whom this is not the case. One reason is likely to be the fact that ACE inhibitors also affect other enzymes, notably kininase, which is involved in the breakdown of vasodilator peptides such as bradykinin and substance P. Of course this does not apply to the receptor antagonists and it is too early to say whether these two drug types have equivalent efficacy.

Advantages

- effective in most patient groups

- safe in most patient types (but see below)

- apparently good 24-hour blood pressure control — high peak/trough ratios for newer agents but methodology controversial

- enhanced well-being reported in some studies — cognitive improvement?

Disadvantages

- first-dose hypotension, especially in sodium- and volume-depleted patients

- irritating cough in 5–20% of patients (with ACE inhibitors only)

- may rarely cause anaphylactoid reactions (probably ACE inhibitors only)

- deterioration in renal function in patients with renovascular disease, owing to altered intrarenal haemodynamics — this can be severe and lead to renal failure. It is possible that the receptor antagonists can cause similar problems but this has yet to be assessed

Alpha₁- adrenergic blockers

Mechanism of action

The principal mode of action of these drugs is the inhibition of noradrenaline-induced vasoconstriction by blocking alpha$_1$-adrenergic receptors in the vascular wall. There may also be some central component, although this may be more important in the prevention of reflex tachycardia than in actually lowering blood pressure.

Advantages

- once-daily dosage for newer compounds

- few contraindications

- neutral or even beneficial metabolic effects, especially on lipid profile

---

Disadvantages

- may cause postural hypotension, particularly 'first dose' effect (less likely with new longer-acting agents)

- can cause tiredness and sedation

- dose may need to be titrated over a broad range

The emphasis on the peripheral vasculature — how appropriate?

It is clear that a wide range of options is available for the prescriber with hypertensive patients. Of course, the drugs can be and very often are used in combinations of two, three or even four, so extending the possibilities even further. Four more recent classes of drugs — calcium channel blockers, angiotensin converting enzyme inhibitors (and angiotensin II receptor antagonists), and alpha-blockers — all have a predominantly peripheral vascular site of action, although the ACE inhibitors and angiotensin receptor blockers probably also have a significant effect on the kidney. The efficacy of these drugs in lowering blood pressure is not in doubt, although long-term outcome data are not yet available. Most patients are also able to tolerate them without great difficulty. Nonetheless, they are associated with significant problems, apart from the fact that in a significant minority of patients blood pressure control is unsatisfactory. To summarize the points already mentioned, as they relate specifically to vascular effects:

- vasodilators are more likely to cause postural hypotension

- they may cause flushing, headache and peripheral oedema

- some can cause reflex sympathetic activation with potentially harmful results

- drugs acting on the renin–angiotensin system may compromise kidney function in the presence of renovascular disease through impairment of glomerular perfusion

It is therefore reasonable to conclude that these drugs are *not* going to be acceptable or adequate for everyone. The older drugs, the thiazides and beta-blockers, will certainly retain first-line status for many if not most clinicians, but reservations are unavoidable in view of metabolic and other unwanted effects.

5. Antihypertensive Drugs Acting on the Sympathetic Nervous System

These drugs, despite their undoubted efficacy, have become increasingly unpopular because of troublesome side-effects and the possibility of rebound hypertension. The older agents are unlikely to be widely used in the future, but newer compounds may combine good efficacy and improved tolerability. The selective imidazoline receptor agonists moxonidine and rilmenidine represent considerable progress in this direction.

These are drugs collectively described as centrally acting antihypertensives or as sympatholytics. In a sense they, too, are vasodilators but their effect is indirect and mediated through their actions on the central regulation of vascular tone. Of course, it is arguable that both alpha- and beta-blockers inhibit sympathetic activity but this is at the level of the target organ, not of the regulatory mechanism. At present few clinicians regard them as first-line drugs in primary hypertension, for reasons that are clarified below.

First-generation drugs: reserpine, methyldopa

Reserpine

Reserpine is one of the oldest recognized therapeutic agents, since it is derived from the root of a shrub, *Rauwolfia serpentina*, which has been used for centuries in traditional Indian and Chinese medicine. The alkaloid reserpine was purified in the 1950s and was used in the pioneering Veterans Administration trial about a decade later. Since then it has virtually disappeared from use in most countries.

Mechanism of action

Reserpine depletes transmitters such as noradrenaline, dopamine and serotonin from central and peripheral neurones. It binds to storage vesicles in nerve endings, damaging their ability to take up and retain the transmitters. These leak into the cytoplasm of the cell and are broken down by enzymes, notably monoamine oxidase. Most of the antihypertensive effect is thought to be centrally mediated. Reserpine reduces both peripheral resistance and cardiac output, as well as heart rate.

Advantages

- long experience of efficacy, including long-term outcome

- simple dosage

- very low cost

Disadvantages

- can cause sedation and depression, sometimes severe
- may cause sodium and water retention

Methyldopa

Methyldopa is an interesting example of a drug designed to work by one mechanism but in fact acting by another. As an analogue of the natural catecholamines it was expected to act as an inhibitor of L-amino acid decarboxylase and therefore inhibit noradrenaline synthesis. Although this does occur, it is not in fact the means by which the drug lowers blood pressure. The compound is converted to the pharmacologically active alpha-methylnoradrenaline, which acts as an agonist for $alpha_2$-receptors in the ventrolateral medulla and inhibits sympathetic outflow (Fig. 15).

Advantages

- long experience of use
- known to be safe in pregnancy

Disdavantages

- sedation, depression, loss of libido

- dry mouth

- sodium and water retention

- may cause parkinsonian syndrome

- hyperprolactinaemia (galactorrhoea, gynaecomastia)

- sometimes causes liver damage, haemolytic anaemia

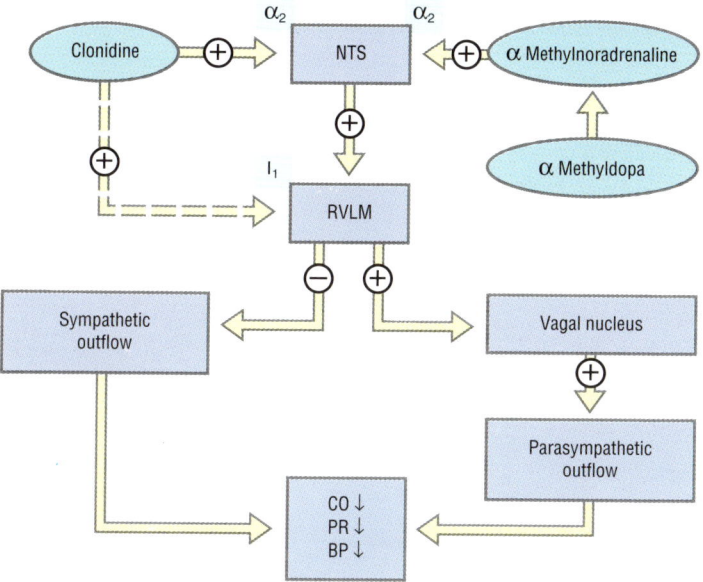

Figure 15
Proposed mechanism of action of clonidine and methyldopa.

Second-generation drugs: clonidine

Clonidine and the much less used *guanabenz* and *guanfacine* are also centrally acting alpha$_2$-agonists, reducing sympathetic activity and therefore both peripheral vascular resistance and cardiac output (Fig. 15). For reasons that will become clear, these drugs are no longer considered of major importance in the treatment of hypertension, except perhaps in the USA. Their efficacy is nonetheless entirely comparable with that of the accepted first-line therapies.

Advantages

- proven efficacy including long-term outcome, equal to current first-line therapies

- no adverse effects on glucose or lipid metabolism, or in asthma

- convenient dosage in modified-release form, or transdermal patch

Disadvantages

- can cause sedation

- dry mouth frequent and sometimes severe

- may cause postural hypotension

- may cause sodium retention

- sexual dysfunction in significant minority of men

- rebound hypertension — much less likely with modified-release formulations or patches, but probably the single most important reason for neglect of this type of drug

Third-generation drugs: imidazoline agonists (moxonidine, rilmenidine)

The centrally acting antihypertensive drugs are certainly not popular at present, although in some patients their usefulness is undeniable. In terms of drug development, work in this area has been far less active than in, say, the renin–angiotensin system, and this trend shows no signs of significant change. The one exception has been the development of the imidazoline I_1-selective agonists, moxonidine and rilmenidine (Fig. 16). These drugs have been available in some Continental European countries for several years but will be unfamiliar to most clinicians in the UK. One of them — moxonidine — has recently been marketed in the UK; it is not clear whether rilmenidine will also be introduced. In view of the novelty of these drugs compared to all the others so far discussed, they will be considered in some detail.

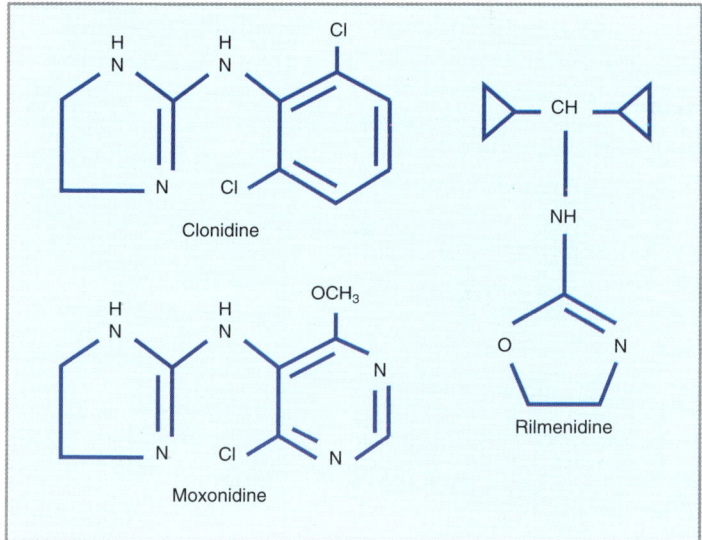

Figure 16
Structures of second- and third-generation centrally acting antihypertensive drugs.

Mechanism of action

At the beginning of this review the rostral ventrolateral medulla was identified as a crucial centre for the regulation of sympathetic outflow and therefore of blood pressure. It was initially believed that the new drugs like moxonidine were, like clonidine, agonists at the alpha$_2$-adrenoceptor at this site in the brain, and that this was the basis of their blood pressure-lowering effect. It is certainly true that there is interaction with the adrenoceptors, but further experiments uncovered a new receptor, the *imidazoline receptor*. As always in pharmacology, there proved to be several subtypes of this receptor and that found in the medulla is now classified as the I_1 -receptor; there is thought to be an endogenous ligand for this receptor, but it has yet to be positively identified. Moxonidine shows up to 70-fold selectivity for the I_1-receptors as compared to the alpha$_2$ - receptor, but the selectivity of rilmenidine may be somewhat less. It now appears that *stimulation of the imidazoline I_1 recep*tor is able to reduce sympathetic activity just as effectively as adrenoceptor stimulation; the receptors are likely to be located on the same neurones in the medulla (Fig. 17). Clonidine may interact with these receptors as well as with the alpha$_2$-adrenoceptors. This is of considerable clinical relevance, especially as regards the adverse effects of the new drugs, since it is generally accepted that *interaction with alpha$_2$ receptors at other sites in the brainstem and in the salivary glands is responsible for the major problems of sedation and dry mouth*. Of course, as usual in pharmacology, selectivity is not absolute and a role for alpha$_2$ -adrenoceptors in the cardiovascular action of the new drugs cannot be excluded.

In experimental models of hypertension moxonidine produces sustained dose-dependent falls in blood pressure. Very importantly, and in contrast to clonidine, *drug withdrawal does not lead to rebound hypertension*. Resting heart rate is little altered, but *exercise-induced tachycardia is reduced*. The hypotensive action also appears to be associated with *regression of left ventricular hypertrophy*. Presumably because of the effect on

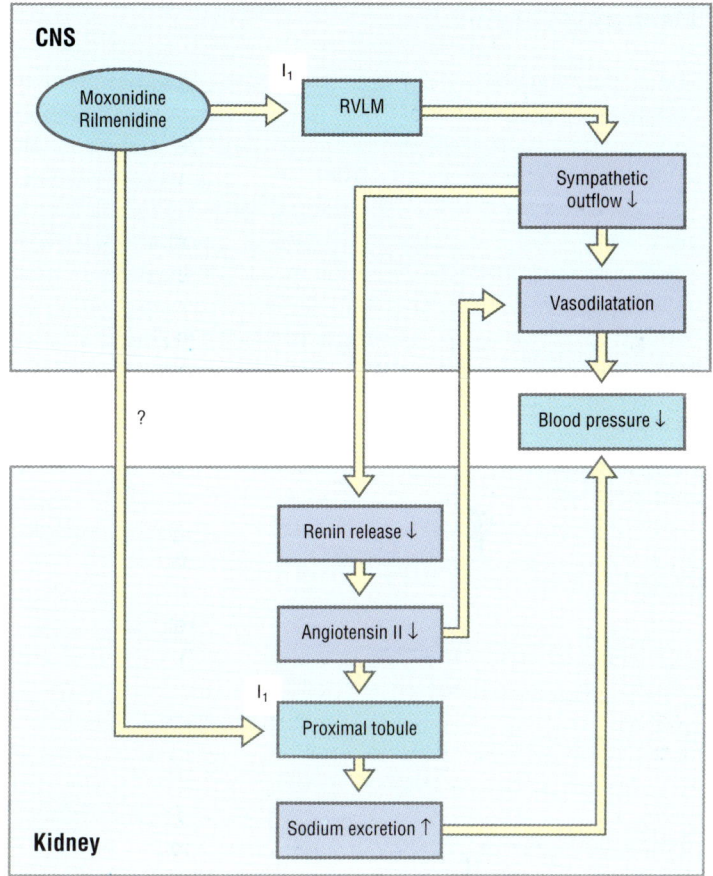

Figure 17
Proposed mechanism of action of the imidazoline I_1 - agonists moxonidine and rilmenidine.

sympathetic activity, moxonidine *reduces plasma renin levels, contributing to natriuresis and diuresis*, although there are no long-term data. There are also believed to be renal I_1 receptors that contribute to this process, which of course is beneficial in terms of blood pressure lowering. A further consequence of sympatholytic activity is *improvement in insulin sensitivity.*

Clinical efficacy

There is now evidence for both moxonidine and rilmenidine, particularly the former, that these drugs are comparable in efficacy to clonidine, and to members of each of the major classes of antihypertensive drugs (atenolol, hydrochlorothiazide, nifedipine modified-release, captopril, and prazosin). Blood pressure control was achieved in 60% or more patients using the drugs as monotherapy. In the majority of patients once-daily dosing was sufficient, but a twice-daily regime may be needed at higher doses. In keeping with its greater affinity for the I_1 receptor the comparable dosage is 0.2–0.4 mg daily for moxonidine compared to 1–2 mg daily for rilmenidine, incidentally indicating a duration of action significantly longer than would be predicted from pharmacokinetic parameters. The following features are characteristically seen, besides blood pressure reduction, and are broadly in keeping with the results from animal experiments:

- reduction in plasma renin activity

- reduced plasma catecholamines

- regression of left ventricular hypertrophy

- no significant change in cardiac output

- heart rate unchanged or slightly reduced

- no evidence that tolerance develops during 1–2 years of therapy

- very significantly, *no rebound hypertension after drug withdrawal* (this may be related to the long duration of action of the drugs, particularly moxonidine)

The drugs are apparently effective in *the elderly* (although studies have not been extensive and there are no specific data on isolated systolic hypertension), in *patients* with *renal impair-*

ment, in whom doses may need adjustment since the kidney is the route of clearance for the drugs, and in *diabetics*. There is little information on patient groups with low renin levels, such as Afro-Caribbeans, and moxonidine is officially contraindicated in the UK in several other patient groups (eg patients with claudication) simply because of lack of clinical data, *not* because there is reason to expect unwanted reactions. Meta-analysis of the clinical trials involving moxonidine suggests that the drug is relatively *more effective in patients with (a) higher baseline blood pressure and (b) higher resting heart rate*. At the moment, information on combinations of the imidazoline agonists with other drugs is rather scanty, but in clinical studies moxonidine has been successfully combined with diuretics and beta-blockers. There is no information at present on the efficacy of the imidazoline agonists in *renovascular hypertension*.

Toxicity and adverse effects

There is *no evidence that either of these drugs is associated with significant hepatic, renal or bone marrow toxicity.* Imidazoline agonists do not have harmful effects in asthma. Other aspects of the drugs' tolerability can be summarized as follows:

- they cause no alterations in levels of plasma electrolytes

- there is no increase in plasma uric acid concentration

- glucose tolerance does not deteriorate

- serum lipids are not adversely affected (there are reports of reductions in low-density cholesterol levels with moxonidine treatment)

- postural hypotension is rare

- significant sodium and water retention has not been reported

Reported unwanted reactions have been few:

- dry mouth: much the most common, up to 15% of patients during early therapy, diminished frequency later (about 2% after 12 months)

- tiredness, lethargy and sedation are less frequent than with the first- and second-generation centrally active drugs

- headache occurs rarely

- dizziness, of unknown mechanism but not directly related to lowered blood pressure, has also been reported

In comparative studies the new drugs were significantly better tolerated than clonidine and at least as well tolerated as any of the established first-line agents. It is too early to say whether sodium retention will prove to be a problem, as it has with earlier centrally acting drugs.

Potential benefits beyond blood pressure lowering?

The clinical history of the imidazoline agonists is rather short, and their place as antihypertensive agents is not fully defined. Even so, preclinical data and results from small clinical studies suggest that they may have useful properties in addition to the lowering of blood pressure, although it must be emphasized that these are *not* substantiated at present and do *not* form any part of the licensed indications of the drugs (of moxonidine specifically, in the case of the UK). The actions include:

- improvement of the metabolic features of the insulin resistance syndrome

- reduction of left ventricular hypertrophy and improvement in coronary microcirculation

- possible antiarrhythmic properties

- some degree of neuroprotection in the presence of ischaemia (probably mediated by I_2 receptors in the cerebral cortex, so that the present I_1-selective drugs may not be optimal for this purpose)

6. Prospects

For most clinicians the concept of stepped care in hypertension is being supplanted by that of individualized treatment, with the characteristics of the patient's hypertension as well as any concurrent disease taken into account. The availability of numerous classes of antihypertensive drugs, with differing mechanisms of action, contributes to the achievement of optimal therapy for each patient.

Individualized therapy for hypertension

Until the 1980s the orthodox approach to the management of hypertension was the 'stepped care' approach, based on initial treatment with either a thiazide diuretic or a beta-blocker, followed by addition of the complementary drug and then other drugs such as hydralazine, clonidine or an alpha-adrenergic blocker such as guanethidine or debrisoquine. The repertoire of better tolerated and generally more effective drugs has now expanded greatly and we understand much more — although not enough — about their metabolic and other potential effects. It is therefore feasible to consider an individualized approach to the management of the hypertensive patient, with other concurrent problems taken into account. This approach is outlined in Table 6. *Please note that this represents the author's personal opinion and may not always conform to the specific product licence of drugs in the UK or other countries.*

An interesting issue, which has perhaps received insufficient attention, can be summarized as follows:

If it is decided that antihypertensive medication is needed, should we:

(a) adopt the same approach as in epilepsy, and use monotherapy until the target blood pressure is reached, or adverse effects limit the dose or cause drug withdrawal; or

(b) use low doses of two drugs in suitable combinations (Table 7) in an attempt to exploit complementary mechanisms of action and minimize adverse reactions?

Most clinicians' practice in fact is closer to the first of these options, even if they have not formally thought about it in detail. Given the pharmacological means at our disposal, this question now requires some debate. There is no 'correct' answer but the second option should at least be considered. The imidazoline agonists can participate in most combinations, a possible exception being co-administration with selective alpha$_1$ -blockers, if there is an analogy with clonidine. However, we need to know more about the role of the drug in combination therapy.

Centrally acting drugs in hypertension — a timely revival?

The decline and indeed virtual disappearance of centrally acting antihypertensive drugs cannot be regarded as surprising. Neither patients nor clinicians found them acceptable, even though they were undoubtedly effective in lowering blood pressure. Many clinicians did, however, regard this as a regrettable

Table 6
Selection of drugs in particular classes of hypertensive patients.

	TD
Black	++
Elderly	++
Angina	+
Cardiac failure	++
Conduction defects	+
Peripheral vascular disease	+
Renovascular disease	+/–
Phaeochromocytoma	+/–
Renal disease	+/–
Diabetes	–?
Raised cholesterol	–
Gout	–
Asthma, COAD	+

gap in the spectrum of treatments available. This has remained so even with the advent of the new and undoubtedly successful drugs. The selective imidazoline receptor agonists clearly go a considerable way towards overcoming the drawbacks of the earlier compounds, although long-term experience with them is still limited and clinical outcome data do not yet exist (of course this is also true of all antihypertensive drugs other than thiazides, beta-blockers and, of course, some earlier centrally acting drugs). They represent a rational choice in several subgroups of hypertensive patients in whom excessive sympathetic activity is likely: notably the *young 'borderline' hypertensive patients* and *patients with features of the insulin resistance syndrome*. Experience with other types of drugs, such as ACE inhibitors, suggests that antihypertensive drugs may also work in patients in whom one would *not* expect success: we are far from proficient at these predictions!

BB	CCB	ACEI, AA	AB	IA
+/−	++	+/−	+	0
−?	+	+	+	+
++	++[1]	+	+	+
−[2]	+/−[3]	++	−?	+
−	−?	+	+	+
−?[4]	++	+	++	0
++	+	−[5]	+	0
++[6]	+	+/−	++[7]	0
+/−	++	++[8]	+	+
−?	+	++	++	+
−, −?[9]	+	++	++	+
+	+	+	+	+
−	+	+[10]	+	+

TD, thiazide diuretics; BB, beta-blockers; CCB, calcium channel blockers; ACEI, angiotensin converting enzyme inhibitors; AA, angiotensin AT_1-receptor antagonists; AB, alpha$_1$-blockers; IA, imidazoline agonists (because of relatively short duration of clinical experience, information incomplete for several conditions).

++	particularly useful, first-choice therapy
+	effective, no significant contraindications
+/−	may not be effective when used alone, although can be useful in combination with other drugs, no contraindications
0	uncertain, information lacking
−?	use with caution if at all
−	avoid

1   Significant differences between different subclasses of CCB
2   Used in certain types of congestive failure on experimental basis
3   as 1
4   Avoid in Raynaud's phenomenon and other small vessel disease, significance in large vessel disease doubtful
5   May be very effective but may also cause serious deterioration in renal function
6   Never to be used without concurrent alpha-blockade
7   Experience with newer drugs (doxazosin, terazosin) limited compared to phentolamine and phenoxybenzamine
8   Complex interactions — differences between subclasses of drugs and according to type of disease
9   Significant differences between subclasses of beta-blockers
10   Few reports of exacerbation of asthma with ACEIs

	TD	BB	CCB	ACEI,AA	AB	IA
TD		+[1]	+	++	−?	+
BB			−?[2]	+	++	+
CCB				++	++	++
ACEI, AA					++	+
AB						−?

Abbreviations as for Table 6
++ particularly rational and useful combination
+   effective combination
−? use with caution
1   widely used but may have adverse metabolic effects in combination
2   significant differences between subclasses of both types of drug

Table 7
Drug combinations in hypertension.

Although it is very probable that other peripherally acting drugs will eventually complement those already in everyday use — for instance, several endothelin antagonists are being developed — effective, safe, and well-tolerated centrally acting drugs are to be welcomed by all clinicians who are involved in the management of hypertension.

Further Reading

This is a very selective list drawn from an overwhelmingly large literature. References relating to imidazoline receptor agonists are listed separately. All the issues raised in this review, and much else, are included in two recent encyclopaedic works:

Laragh J, Brenner, BM,. eds. (1995) *Hypertension: Pathophysiology, Diagnosis, and Management.* 2nd edn (Raven Press: New York).

Swales JD, ed. (1994) *Textbook of Hypertension* (Blackwell Scientific Publications: Oxford).

A less conventional but very useful and up-to-date approach is to be found in the following:

Hollenberg NK, ed. (1995) Atlas of Heart Diseases, volume 1. *Hypertension: Mechanisms and Therapy.* (Current Medicine: Philadelphia).

General references

Anderson EA, Sinkey CA, Lawton WJ, Mark AL (1989) Elevated sympathetic nerve activity in borderline hypertensive humans: evidence from direct intra-neuronal recordings, *Hypertension* **14**:177–83.

Arauz-Pacheco C, Lender D, Snell PG, Huet B, Ramirez LC, Breen L, Mora P, Raskin P (1996) Relationship between insulin sensitivity, hyperinsulinemia, and insulin mediated sympathetic activation in normotensive and hypertensive subjects, *Am J Hypertens* **9**:1172–8.

Bönner G (1994) Hyperinsulinemia, insulin resistance, and hypertension. *J Cardiovasc Pharmacol* **24** (suppl 2):S39–S49.

Chalmers J (1993) The place of combination therapy in the treatment of hypertension in 1993, *Clin Exp Hypertens* **15**:1299–313.

de Courten M, Zimmet P, Hodge A, Collins V, Nicolson M, Staten M, Dowse G, Alberti KGGM (1997) Hyperleptinaemia: the missing link in the metabolic syndrome? *Diabet Med* **14**:200-8.

Epstein M, Bakris G (1996) Newer approaches to antihypertensive therapy. Use of fixed-dose combination therapy, *Arch Int Med* **156**:1969–78.

Esler MD, Lambert GW, Ferrier CK, Kaye DM, Wallin BG, Kalff V, Kelly MJ, Jennings GL (1995) Central nervous system noradrenergic control of sympathetic outflow in normotensive and hypertensive humans, *Clin Exp Hypertens* **17**:409–23.

Facchini FS, Toohs RA, Reaven GM (1996) Enhanced sympathetic nervous system activity. The linchpin between insulin resistance, hyperinsulinemia, and heart rate, *Am J Hypertens* **9**:1013–17.

Firth JD, Raine AEG, Ledingham JGG (1990) The mechanism of pressure-natriuresis, *J Hypertens*, **8**:97–104.

Folkow B (1989) Sympathetic nervous control of blood pressure: role in primary hypertension, *Am J Hypertens* **2** (suppl):103S–111S.

Folkow B (1993) Early structural changes in hypertension: pathophysiology and clinical consequences, *J Cardiovasc Pharmacol* **22** (suppl 1):S1–S6.

Gudbjörnsdóttir S, Lönnroth P, Sverissdóttir YB, Wallin BG, Elam M (1996) Sympathetic nerve activity and insulin in obese normotensive and hypertensive men, *Hypertension* **27**:276–80.

Guyton AC (1987) Renal function curve — a key to understanding the pathogenesis of hypertension, *Hypertension* **10**:1–6.

Haddy FJ, Pamnani MB (1995) Role of dietary salt in hypertension, *J Am Coll Nutr* **14**:428–38.

Hall JE, Zappe DH, Alonso-Garcia M, Granger JP, Brands MW, Kassab SE (1996) Mechanisms of obesity-induced hypertension, *News Physiol Sci* **11**:255–61.

Hall JE, Brands MW, Shek EW (1996) Central role of the kidney and abnormal fluid volume control in hypertension, *J Hum Hypertens* **10**:633–39.

Hansen J, Victor RG (1994) Direct measurement of sympathetic activity: new insights into disordered blood pressure regulation in chronic renal failure, *Current Opin Nephrol Hypertens* **3**:636–43.

Hollenberg NK (1996) Genes, hypertension and intermediate phenotypes, *Curr Opin Cardiol* **11**: 457–63.

Hopkins PN, Hunt SC, Wu LL, Williams GH, Williams RR (1996) Hypertension, dyslipidemia, and insulin resistance: links in a chain or spokes on a wheel? *Curr Opin Lipidol* **7**:241–53.

Ikeda T, Gomi T, Hirawa N, Sakurai J, Yoshikawa N (1996) Improvement of insulin sensitivity contributes to blood pressure reduction after weight loss in hypertensive subjects with obesity. *Hypertension* **27**:1180–86.

Julius S, Jamerson K (1994) Sympathetics, insulin resistance and coronary risk in hypertension, *J Hypertens* **12**:495–502.

Kotchen TA, Kotchen JM, O'Shaughnessy IM (1996) Insulin and hypertensive cardiovascular disease, *Curr Opin Cardiol* **11**:483–9.

Krönig BB, Kirch W, Welzel D, Weidinger G (1997) Different concepts in first-line treatment of essential hypertension. Comparison of a low-dose reserpine–thiazide combination with nitrendipine monotherapy, *Hypertension* **29**:651–8.

Landsberg L (1994) Pathophysiology of obesity-related hypertension: role of insulin and the sympathetic nervous system, *J Cardiovasc Pharmacol* **23** (suppl 1):S1–S8.

Lever AF, Harrap SB (1992) Essential hypertension: a disorder of growth with origins in childhood, *J Hypertens* **10**:101–20.

Lifton RP (1995) Genetic determinants of human hypertension, *Proc Nat Acad Sci USA* **92**:8545–51.

Lifton RP (1996) Molecular genetics of human blood pressure variation, *Science* **272**:676–80.

Mao AO, Gibbons GH (1994) New insights on renovascular hypertension, *Curr Opin Cardiol* **9**:598–605.

Masuo K, Mikami H, Ogihara T, Tuck ML (1997) Sympathetic nerve hyperactivity precedes hyperinsulinemia and blood pressure elevation in a young, nonobese Japanese population, *Am J Hypertens* **10**:77–83.

Mediratta S, Fozailoff A, Frishman WH (1995) Insulin resistance in systemic hypertension: pharmacotherapeutic implications, *J Clin Pharmacol* **35**:943–56.

Nava E, Lüscher TF (1995) Endothelium-derived vasoactive factors in hypertension: nitric oxide and endothelin, *J Hypertens* **13** (suppl):S39–S48.

Noll G, Wenzel RR, Schneider M, Oesch V, Binggeli C, Shaw S, Weidmann P, Lüscher TF (1996) Increased activation of sympathetic nervous system and endothelin by mental stress in normotensive offspring of hypertensive parents, *Circulation* **93**:866–9.

Omvik P, Tarazi RC, Bravo EL (1980) Regulation of sodium balance in hypertension, *Hypertension* **2**:515–23.

Reaven GM, Lithell H, Landsberg L (1996) Hypertension and associated metabolic abnormalities — the role of insulin resistance and the sympathoadrenal system, *N Engl J Med* **334**:374–81.

Reaven GM (1995) Pathophysiology of insulin resistance in human disease, *Physiol Rev* **75**:473–87.

Robertson JIS (1994) Guidelines for the treatment of hypertension: a critical review, *Cardiovas Drugs Ther* **8**:665–72.

Sanders PW (1996) Salt-sensitive hypertension: lessons from animal models, *Am J Kidney Dis* **28**:775–82.

Schiffrin EL (1995) Endothelin: potential role in hypertension and vascular hypertrophy, *Hypertension* **25**:1135–43.

Sever PS, Poulter NS (1989) A hypothesis for the pathogenesis of essential hypertension: the initiating factors, *J Hypertens* **7** (suppl):S9–S12.

Spyer KM (1990) CNS organization of reflex circulatory control. In: Loewy AD, Spyer KM, eds, *Central Regulation of Autonomic Functions* (Oxford University Press: New York) 168–88.

Staessen JA, Poulter NR, Fletcher AE, Markowe HL, Marmot MG, Shipley MJ, Bulpitt CJ (1994) Psycho-emotional stress and salt intake may interact to raise blood pressure, *J Cardiovas Risk* **1**:45–51.

Staessen JA, Bienaszewski L, Pardaens K, Petrov V, Thijs L, Fagard R (1996) Life style as a blood pressure determinant, *J R Soc Med* **89**:484–9.

Taddei S, Viridis A, Mattei P, Duranti P, Favilla S, Salvetti A (1994) Vascular renin–angiotensin system and sympathetic nervous system activity in human hypertension, *J Cardiovasc Pharmacol* **23** (suppl 1):S9–S14.

van Paasen P, de Zeeuw D, Navis G, de Jong PE (1996) Does the renin–angiotensin system determine the renal and systemic hemodynamic response to sodium in patients with essential hypertension? *Hypertension* **27**:202–8.

Weidmann P, Bohlen L, de Courten M (1995) Insulin resistance and hyperinsulinemia in hypertension, *J Hypertens* **13** (suppl):S65–S72.

Weinberger MH (1996) Salt sensitivity of blood pressure in humans, *Hypertension* **27** (part 2): 481–90.

Imidazoline receptors and imidazoline agonists

Much of the information in this area has been published in sponsored journal supplements and special issues:

American Journal of Hypertension (1992) **5** (4) Supplement

Annals of the New York Academy of Sciences (1995) **763**

Cardiovascular Drugs and Therapy (1994) **8** Supplement 1

Cardiovascular Drugs and Therapy (1996) **10** Supplement 1

Cardiovascular Risk Factors (1994) **5** Supplement 1

Journal of Cardiovascular Pharmacology (1992) **20** Supplement 4

Journal of Cardiovascular Pharmacology (1994) **24** Supplement 1

Journal of Cardiovascular Pharmacology (1996) **27** Supplement 3

Journal of Hypertension (1997) **15** Supplement 1

as well as a monograph:

van Zwieten PA, Hamilton CA, Julius S, Brichard BNC eds. (1996) The I_1-imidazoline Agonist Moxonidine: a New Antihypertensive (Royal Society of Medicine Press: London).

In addition, the following individual papers and reviews are relevant:

Chan CKS, Head GA (1996) Relative importance of central imidazoline receptors for the antihypertensive effects of moxonidine and rilmenidine, J Hypertens **14**:855–64.

Chrisp P, Faulds D (1992) Moxonidine. A review of its pharmacology, and therapeutic use in essential hypertension, Drugs **44**:993–1012.

Küppers HE, Jäger BA, Luszik JH, Gräve MA, Hughes PR, Kaan EC (1997) Placebo-controlled comparison of the efficacy and tolerability of once-daily moxonidine and enalapril in mild-to-moderate essential hypertension, J Hypertens **15**:93-97.

Reid JL (1996) New therapeutic agents for hypertension, Br J Clin Pharmacol **42**:37–41.

Rupp H, Jacob R (1995) Excess catecholamines and the metabolic syndrome: should central imidazoline receptors be a therapeutic target? Med Hypotheses **44**:217–25.

Urban R, Szabo B, Starke K (1995) Involvement of alpha$_2$ - adrenoceptors in the cardiovascular effects of moxonidine, *Eur J Pharmacol* **282**:19–28.

Yu A, Frishman WH (1996) Imidazoline receptor agonist drugs: a new approach to the treatment of systemic hypertension, *J Clin Pharmacol* **36**:98–111.

van Zwieten PA (1997) Central imidazoline (I$_1$) receptors as targets of centrally acting antihypertensives: moxonidine and rilmenidine, *J Hypertens* **15**:117–25.

Index

Page numbers in *italic* refer to the illustrations